Mediterranean Diet Recipes

50 Fresh Mediterranean Diet Recipes for Delicious Weight Loss

Benjamin Tideas

CONTENTS

INTRODUCTION

Nice job picking up this convenient cookbook to assist with your weight loss goals on the Mediterranean Diet. I think you'll find many different options that are delicious, but still legal to your diet.

I won't impede your journey to the tasty Salads, Soups, Pasta, and Wraps you'll find in this book. Remember to watch portion sizes, as with any diet – even delicious recipes can add pounds if you eat too much.

Please enjoy the recipes with the handy quick content links above, and don't forget to pick up your free report here:
http://www.plaid-enterprises.com/mediterranean

Bon Appetit!

Benjamin Tideas

SALADS

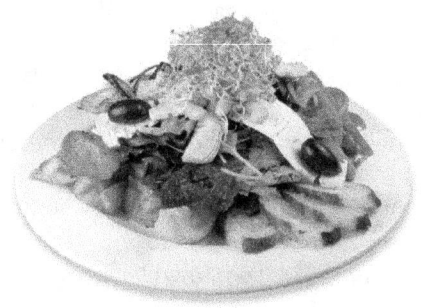

Mediterranean Greek Salad

Ingredients
18 cups torn romaine (2 bunches)
1 cup crumbled feta cheese
1/2 cup pitted Greek olives
1/2 cup julienned roasted sweet red peppers
1 small red onion, thinly sliced
1 cup cherry tomatoes, sliced
1 medium cucumber, sliced

Toss ingredients in a large salad bowl and serve with low-fat Greek Dressing. Season with cracked peppercorns.

Classic Greek Salad

Ingredients
Freshly ground pepper
5 Persian cucumbers
Kosher salt
Grated zest and juice of 1 lemon
1 teaspoon dried oregano
1 cup kalamata olives, halved and pitted
1 teaspoon honey
1 small red onion, halved and thinly sliced
12 to 14 small vine-ripened tomatoes, quartered
14 -ounce block Greek feta cheese, packed in brine
¼ cup red wine vinegar
¼ cup extra-virgin olive oil, plus more for drizzling
Fresh oregano leaves, for topping (optional)

Soak the red onion in a bowl of heavily salted ice water for 15 minutes. Whisk the vinegar, lemon zest and juice, honey, dried oregano, 1/2 teaspoon salt and 1/4 teaspoon pepper in a large bowl. Whisk in the olive oil in a slow, steady stream until emulsified. Add the tomatoes and olives and toss.

Peel the cucumbers, leaving alternating strips of green peel. Trim the ends, halve lengthwise and slice crosswise, about 1/2 inch thick; add to the bowl with the tomatoes. Drain the red onion, add to the bowl and toss.

Drain the feta and slice horizontally into 4 even rectangles. Divide the salad among plates. Top with the feta and oregano; drizzle with olive oil and season with pepper.

Classic Greek Salad Topped with Grilled Calamari Skewers

Ingredients
20 wooden skewers
10 small whole calamari, cleaned, tentacles removed
1/2 cup extra-virgin olive oil, plus more for grilling
1/4 cup red wine vinegar
4 garlic cloves, chopped
1 tablespoon dried oregano
1 tablespoon fresh oregano
1 tablespoon fresh thyme leaves
1 lemon, juiced
Kosher salt and freshly ground black pepper
4 tomatoes, seeded and cut into chunks
1 medium red onion, sliced thin
1 medium cucumber, sliced thin
1/2 pound feta cheese, crumbled
1/2 cup kalamata olives, pitted
1 head romaine lettuce, torn into bite size pieces
Lemon wedges, for garnish
Fresh oregano leaves, for garnish

Soak the 20 wooden skewers in water for about 20 minutes.
Rinse the calamari tubes and then, pat dry.
Split the bodies from top to bottom so that you have 2 triangular pieces.
Thread a soaked skewer through the length of each piece.
Put the skewers on a platter and set aside.

To make the vinaigrette, whisk together the oil, vinegar, garlic, dried and fresh oregano, thyme and lemon juice; season with salt and pepper.

Pour 1/2 of the vinaigrette over the calamari; set the other 1/2 aside while you make the salad.

In a large bowl, add the tomatoes, onion, cucumber, cheese, olives, and romaine. Pour the remaining vinaigrette over the salad and toss to combine. Let marinate while you grill the calamari.

Heat the grill or a grill pan and oil it lightly. Grill the calamari for 2 minutes on each side, no longer or they will be tough. To serve, put the salad onto a large platter and top it with the calamari skewers. Garnish with fresh oregano leaves and lemon wedges.

Greek Dinner Salad

Ingredients
Kosher salt and freshly ground pepper
2 tablespoons red wine vinegar
1 small clove garlic, minced
2 romaine lettuce hearts, thinly sliced crosswise
1 cup mixed fresh herbs (parsley, dill, mint and/or oregano)
1 cup crumbled feta cheese
1 pint cherry tomatoes, halved
2 large cucumbers, peeled, seeded and cut into chunks
12 stuffed grape leaves (from the deli counter)
1/2 small red onion, thinly sliced
1/3 cup extra-virgin olive oil
1 cup pepperoncini and/or kalamata olives, plus 1 tablespoon brine from the jar

Soak the onion in a small bowl of ice water for about 5 minutes. Make the dressing: Whisk the vinegar, pepperoncini or olive brine, garlic, 1/2 teaspoon salt and 1/4 teaspoon pepper in a large bowl. Whisk in the olive oil in a slow stream until blended.

Drain the onion and add to the bowl with the dressing. Add the lettuce, herbs, tomatoes and cucumbers and toss to combine. Season with salt and pepper. Divide among bowls and top with the pepperoncini and/or olives, feta and stuffed grape leaves.

Antipasti Dinner Salad

Ingredients
Freshly ground pepper
Kosher salt
1/2 cup extra-virgin olive oil, plus more for drizzling
1 small head radicchio, thinly sliced
2 large cloves garlic, smashed
2 romaine lettuce hearts, halved lengthwise
2 tablespoons red wine vinegar
3 stalks celery, thinly sliced
8 slices rustic Italian bread
6 ounces deli-sliced hard salami or soppressata, cut into strips
8 ounces small mozzarella balls (bocconcini), halved
10 to 15 fresh basil leaves, sliced if large
20 cured black olives (such as kalamata or nicoise), pitted and halved

Heat 3 tablespoons of olive oil in a large skillet over medium heat. Add the garlic and cook until fragrant for about 1 minute. Increase the heat to high and add the bread in batches. Toast until golden on both sides. Set aside and season with salt.

Whisk the vinegar, the remaining 5 tablespoons oil, 1/2 teaspoon salt and pepper to taste in a large bowl. Add the radicchio, celery, salami, basil, mozzarella and olives; toss to coat.

Place 1 romaine half on each plate. Drizzle with olive oil and season with salt and pepper. Spoon the salad onto each wedge, drizzling any remaining dressing on top; serve with the toasts.

Mediterranean Basmati Salad

Ingredients
2 sun-dried tomatoes, packed without oil
1 tablespoon olive oil
2 tablespoons dried currants
2 tablespoons chopped fresh mint
1/4 teaspoon black pepper
1/4 cup hot water
1/2 teaspoon salt
1 1/4 cups uncooked basmati rice
2/3 cup (2.5 ounces) feta cheese, crumbled
2 cups water

Combine tomatoes and water in a small bowl and let stand for 10 minutes. Drain and chop; set aside.

Place rice in a large bowl and cover with water to 2 inches above rice. Soak for 30 minutes while stirring occasionally. Drain and rinse.

Combine rice and 2 cups water in a small saucepan; stir in salt. Boil over medium-high heat for 5 minutes or until water level falls just below rice, stirring frequently. Cover, reduce heat to low, and cook 10 minutes. Remove from heat; let stand, covered, 10 minutes.

Spoon rice into a bowl; cool completely and fluff with a fork. Stir in tomatoes, feta, and next 4 ingredients (through pepper); toss well to combine. Sprinkle with pine nuts.

Mediterranean Crispy Chickpea Salad

Ingredients
1 tablespoon finely chopped fresh oregano
1 clove garlic, minced
¼ teaspoon pepper
¼ small red onion, chopped (about 3 Tbsp.)
½ teaspoon salt
½ teaspoon ground cumin
½ small English cucumber, chopped (about 1 cup)
½ cup crumbled feta, optional
½ cup coarsely chopped pitted kalamata or green olives
1 15.5-oz. can chickpeas, drained and rinsed
2 tablespoons red wine vinegar
3 tablespoons extra-virgin olive oil
3 cups chopped romaine, from 1 large heart

In a medium bowl, whisk together 1 tbsp oil, cumin and 1/4 tsp. salt. Add chickpeas, stirring to coat. In a medium nonstick skillet, cook chickpea mixture over medium-high heat, stirring occasionally, until chickpeas are golden brown and slightly crisp, 4 to 5 minutes. Add garlic and cook, stirring, until golden and fragrant, 30 seconds. Transfer to a plate.

In a large bowl, whisk together vinegar, remaining 2 Tbsp. oil, oregano and 1/4 tsp. each salt and pepper. Add romaine, cucumber, onion, chickpeas, olives and feta, if desired. Toss until well coated and serve.

Mediterranean Salad

Ingredients
Salt and pepper
Zest of 1 lemon
2 teaspoons chopped fresh oregano, or 1 1/4 tsp. dried
2 tablespoons chopped fresh mint leaves, or 1 1/4 tsp. dried
6 tablespoons fresh lemon juice
1 small bulb fennel, quartered, cored, sliced very thin
2 cucumbers, cut into 1-inch pieces
1 ½ teaspoons whole fennel seeds
1 15.5 oz. can chickpeas, drained and rinsed
2/3 cup extra-virgin olive oil
1 14-oz. can hearts of palm, drained, cut into 1-inch pieces
1 12-oz. can artichoke hearts, drained and quartered
6 ounces feta, broken into chunks
2/3 cup pitted kalamata olives
1 12-oz. jar roasted red peppers, drained, cut into strips
4 cups chopped romaine lettuce

Place the fennel seeds in a medium skillet over medium heat and cook, tossing, until fragrant for 2 to 3 minutes. Add chickpeas and 1 tbsp. oil. Season it with salt and sauté until warmed through, about 2 minutes. Transfer to a bowl to cool. In a separate large bowl, whisk remaining oil with lemon zest and lemon juice, oregano and mint. Season it with salt and pepper.

Toss lettuce in a third bowl with 2 tbsp. dressing. Arrange lettuce on a large platter. In the same bowl, toss chickpea mixture with 2 tbsp. dressing. On top of lettuce, arrange each of remaining ingredients in rows. Serve with remaining dressing on the side.

Mediterranean Couscous and Lentil Salad

Ingredients
1 cup dried lentils
1 (14-ounce) can fat-free, less-sodium chicken broth
1 1/2 cups uncooked couscous
1 cup diced red bell pepper
1 cup chopped fresh mint
1/2 cup chopped fresh parsley
1/2 cup chopped green onions
1/2 cup fresh lemon juice
1/4 cup olive oil
1 tablespoon Dijon mustard
1 1/2 teaspoons minced garlic
1/2 teaspoon black pepper
1 cup (4 ounces) crumbled feta cheese

Place lentils in a large saucepan; cover with water 2 inches above lentils. Bring to a boil; cover, reduce heat, and simmer 25 to 30 minutes or until tender. Drain well; cool.

Bring broth to a boil in a medium saucepan; gradually stir in couscous. Remove from heat; cover and let stand 5 minutes. Fluff with a fork.

Combine lentils, couscous, bell pepper, and next 3 ingredients in a large bowl; stir gently.

Combine lemon juice and next 4 ingredients in a small bowl. Pour lemon juice mixture over couscous mixture; stir gently. Stir in cheese.

Mediterranean Carrot Salad

Ingredients
2 cloves finely chopped garlic
1/4 cup fresh lemon juice
1/4 cup extra-virgin olive oil
2 teaspoons sugar
1/2 teaspoon dried basil
1/4 teaspoon dried oregano
1 pound peeled carrots
3/4 cup brine-cured, pitted Mediterranean olives
1/2 cup chopped fresh Italian parsley
1/2 cup crumbled feta

Combine 2 cloves finely chopped garlic with 2 tbsp. in a very hot water in a medium bowl and set aside for 5 minutes. Then whisk in 1/4 cup fresh lemon juice, 1/4 cup extra-virgin olive oil, 2 tsp. sugar, 1/2 tsp. dried basil, 1/4 tsp. dried oregano, and salt and pepper to taste until blended.

Fold in 1 lb. peeled carrots, sliced diagonally into 1/8-inch-thick slices, and 3/4 cup brine-cured, pitted Mediterranean olives, drained and sliced in half. Cover and refrigerate for at least 15 minutes. Fold in 1/2 cup chopped fresh Italian parsley and top with 1/2 cup crumbled feta when ready to serve.

SOUP

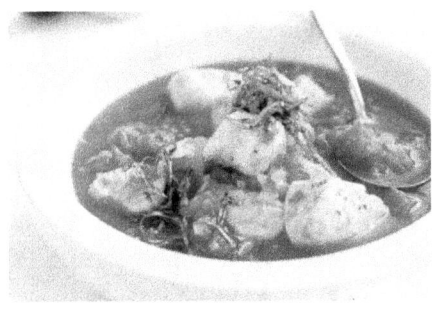

Mediterranean Vegetable soup

Ingredients
1 tablespoon olive oil
1 onion, diced
1 carrot, halved lengthwise and sliced
2 stalks celery, sliced
3 cloves garlic, minced
2 cups chicken or beef broth
2 cups water
1 can (14 1/2 ounces) diced tomatoes, not drained
1 tablespoon fresh basil, chopped
1/4 teaspoon oregano
salt and pepper to taste
1 15 oz. can cannellini or white beans, drained and rinsed
1 cup pasta bows (or other small pasta)
Parmesan cheese (optional)
1 small head escarole (optional)

Heat the oil in a heavy saucepan over medium heat. Add the onion, carrot and celery, and sauté until tender, about 5 minutes. Add the garlic, broth, water, tomatoes, basil, oregano, salt, pepper, and beans.

Bring to a boil, reduce heat and simmer for 10 minutes. If escarole is being used, wash and tear into 2 inch pieces and add to soup 15 minutes before soup is done, or at the same time as the pasta.

Add the pasta bows and cook 10-15 minutes, stirring occasionally until the pasta is cooked and the escarole is tender.
Serve sprinkled with Parmesan cheese.

Mediterranean Fish Soup

Ingredients
¼ tsp. red pepper flakes
¼ c. white wine
½ tsp. spearmint
½ tsp. basil
½ to 1 tsp. salt
1 (8 oz.) bottle clam juice
1 to 1 ½ lb. fish fillets
1 med. onion, diced
1 tsp. garlic
1 tsp. black pepper
1 carrot, diced
2 tbsp. olive oil
2 med. diced potatoes
3 stalks celery, diced
26 oz. canned tomatoes, chopped
Dash Pernod, optional

Place the potatoes in the pot with clam juice and/or water to cover. Bring to a boil, reduce heat and simmer until potatoes are tender. In second pot, sauté the onion and garlic in the olive oil. Add the spices and sauté for 2 minutes.

Add the celery, carrots, and wine. Cook all until tender. Add the chopped tomatoes, Pernod, potatoes, and their liquid. Taste and add salt. Chop fish bite sized, removing bones. Add to soup. Heat through until fish is cooked.

Mediterranean Style Fish Soup

Ingredients
¼ c. olive oil
¼ to ½ c. pesto sauce
½ tsp. basil
½ tsp. thyme
½ tsp. oregano
1 c. fresh parsley, chopped
1 lg. bay leaf
2 c. sliced onions
2 qts. chicken broth or fish stock
2 lbs. fresh and/or canned and/or frozen fish/shrimp/clams, chunked
8 cloves garlic, unpeeled, roughly chopped
28 oz. can whole tomatoes with liquid
Salt and pepper to taste

Sauté the onions in oil 8-10 minutes until tender, but not brown. Add the garlic, tomato, herbs. Simmer for 3-4 minutes. Pour in liquid. Boil slowly, lightly covered for 45 minutes.

Strain, degrease, if desired, return liquid in pan. Return to boil. Add the raw seafood first. Simmer until opaque. Add any precooked seafood. Stir until heated through. Ladle into warm bowls and top with dollop of pesto and parsley. Freezes nicely.

Mussel Soup In The Mediterranean Style

Ingredients
¼ tsp. saffron threads, or 1 sm. hot red pepper
½ lb. ripe red plum tomatoes, approximately
1 lg. leek
1 salted anchovy or 4 canned anchovy filets
1 bunch parsley, minced
2 qts. fresh mussels
2 c. white wine
2 tbsp. plus approximately 1/4 c. olive oil
3 cloves garlic
6 thin slices crusty country-style bread
Salt and fresh ground pepper to taste

Rinse the mussels under running water, discarding any that are open. Place in a soup kettle with white wine. Bring to a fast boil over medium-high heat and steam until mussels open. Remove mussels from broth, being careful not to pick up sandy sediment. Strain the broth carefully through a colander lined with cheesecloth into a measuring cup. Add water to make 4 cups liquid.

Rinse out soup kettle. Clean and slice the leek thinly and sauté it in 2 tablespoons of oil over gentle heat until leek has softened. If using salted anchovy, split it in half and rinse under running water to rid it of salt. Pull away the bones. Pat anchovy dry.

Mash 2 garlic cloves and mince with anchovy and half the parsley. Add to leek and sauté until garlic starts to turn golden. Roughly chop tomatoes. Add to soup kettle with mussel broth and either saffron threads or hot pepper.

Let simmer, partly covered, 10 minutes. Taste for seasoning and add salt and pepper to taste. While liquid is simmering, remove the empty half shell from each mussel, leaving only the shell half that has the mussel in it. Discard empty shells.

Add the mussels in shells to the simmering broth, and let warm to serving temperature. While broth is warming, toast the bread slices on both sides. When bread is toasted, cut remaining clove of garlic and rub over bread. Drizzle a little of the remaining olive oil over each slice. Place a bread slice in bottom of each soup bowl.

When ready to serve, place a ladleful of mussels in each bowl on top of the sliced bread. Pour broth over, discarding hot pepper if used. Sprinkle with minced parsley and serve immediately.

Mediterranean Minestrone

Ingredients
¼ tsp. garlic powder
¼ c. chopped parsley
½ tsp. black pepper
1 (10 oz.) pkg. frozen peas
1 (15 oz.) can tomato sauce
1 (20 oz.) can white or red kidney beans
1 (28 oz.) can tomatoes
2 lbs. beef soup bone (optional)
2 med. onions, quartered
2 tbsp. salt
2 c. sliced carrots
2 tsp. basil, crushed
2 bay leaves
2 c. sliced celery
2 (8 oz.) pkg. frozen Italian green beans
3 lbs. beef, sliced
4 c. uncooked macaroni
4 qts. water
Grated Parmesan

Place the meat and bones in 8 or 10 quarts soup kettle. Add water and bring it to a boil. Add the tomatoes, sauce, onions and seasonings. Cover and simmer for 1 ½ hours.

Add carrots and celery, simmer ½ hour or until meat is tender. Remove the meat and bones, discard the bones and fat. Cut the meat in bite size pieces and return to soup.

Heat the soup to a boiling point, add the uncooked macaroni, green beans, and peas. Cook for 15 to 20 minutes until macaroni is tender. Stir in kidney beans and heat to bubbling. Serve with Parmesan cheese. Makes 6 quarts. May be frozen, leave 1 inch at top of container.

Mediterranean Stew

Ingredients
¼ tsp. pepper
½ c. elbow macaroni
1 tbsp. butter
1 tsp. Worcestershire sauce
1 c. grated raw carrots
2 lbs. ground beef
2 tbsp. minced onions
2 c. sliced celery
2 tbsp. parsley
2 c. diced potatoes
2 tbsp. salt
4 lbs. canned tomatoes
4 cans consommé beef broth (soup)

Small beans, baked beans, lima beans - anything may be added. Cook several hours and it is a meal in itself with salad and rolls.

Mediterranean Chickpea, Tomato, and Pasta Soup

Ingredients
2 teaspoons olive oil
1 cup diced onion
1 1/2 cups water
1 (16-ounce) can fat-free, less-sodium chicken broth
1/2 teaspoon ground cumin
1/4 teaspoon ground cinnamon
1/4 teaspoon black pepper
1 (15 1/2-ounce) can chickpeas (garbanzo beans), drained
1 (14.5-ounce) can diced tomatoes, undrained
1/2 cup uncooked ditalini (very short tube-shaped macaroni)
2 tablespoons chopped fresh parsley

Heat the olive oil in a large saucepan over medium-high heat. Add the onion, and sauté for 3 minutes or until tender. Add the water and the next 6 ingredients (water through tomatoes).

Bring mixture to a boil; cover, reduce heat, and simmer 5 minutes, stirring occasionally. Add the pasta, and cook 9 minutes or until pasta is tender. Stir in chopped parsley.

Greek-Style Clam Soup

Ingredients
1/3 cup chopped fresh parsley
¼ cup chopped fresh oregano
½ teaspoon salt
1 cup chopped onion
1 cup dry white wine
2 (8-ounce) bottles clam juice
2 tablespoons fresh lemon juice
2 tablespoons olive oil
3 cups hot cooked orzo (about 1 1/2 cups uncooked rice-shaped pasta)
3 cups chopped seeded peeled tomato
3 cups water
5 garlic cloves, minced
6 tablespoons crumbled feta cheese
30 littleneck clams, scrubbed (about 2 pounds)

Heat the oil in a large Dutch oven over medium-high heat. Add the onion, salt, and garlic; sauté for 4 minutes. Stir in tomato; cook 8 minutes, stirring occasionally. Stir in 3 cups water, wine, and clam juice and bring to a boil. Reduce heat, and simmer 6 minutes.

Add the clams to the pan. Cover and cook for 10 minutes or until clams open; discard any unopened shells. Remove from heat. Stir in parsley, oregano, and lemon juice. Place ½ cup pasta in each of 6 soup bowls; ladle 5 clams and about 1 cup broth over each serving. Top each serving with 1 tablespoon cheese.

Mediterranean Chicken Soup

Ingredients
1 cup kalamata olives, pitted and chopped
1 large yellow onion, quartered
1 cup fresh flat-leaf parsley leaves, roughly chopped
1 teaspoon whole black peppercorns
1 3 1/2- to 4-pound chicken
1 10-ounce box couscous
1 15-ounce can chickpeas, drained and rinsed
2 1/2 teaspoons kosher salt
4 celery stalks
6 carrots, peeled

Rinse the chicken inside and out and pat it dry with paper towel. Place the chicken in a large pot.

Cut 3 of the carrots and 2 of the celery stalks into 1-inch pieces. Quarter the onion. Add the cut vegetables to the pot with the salt, peppercorns, and enough cold water to cover (about 8 cups). Bring to a boil. Reduce heat and simmer, skimming any foam that rises to the top, until the chicken is cooked through, about 30 minutes. Transfer the chicken to a bowl and let cool.

Strain the broth, discarding the vegetables. Return the broth to the pot.

Thinly slice the remaining carrots and celery. Add them to the broth and simmer until tender, about 10 minutes.

While the soup simmers, cook the couscous according to the package directions. Add the olives and parsley to the couscous and divide among bowls.

When the chicken is cool enough to handle, shred the meat and add it to the soup. Stir in the chickpeas. Ladle the soup over the couscous. Serve with lemon wedges.

Mediterranean Three Bean Soup

Ingredients
Pepper to taste
1 tsp. marjoram
1 bay leaf
1 sm. onion, chopped fine
1 tsp. thyme
1 can chick peas
1 can stewed tomatoes
1 can kidney beans
1 can northern beans
2 lg. cloves garlic, minced
2 stalks celery, chopped fine
4 c. chicken or beef broth

Mix all together; bring to a boil, lower heat and simmer for 20-30 minutes.

PASTA

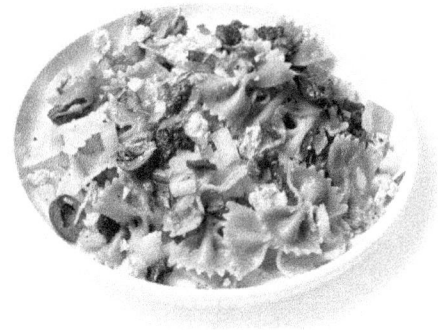

Mediterranean Pasta with Artichokes, Olives, and Tomatoes

Ingredients
Coarse salt and ground pepper
¼ cup grated Parmesan cheese, plus more serving
1/3 cup pitted kalamata olives, quartered lengthwise
½ cup fresh basil leaves, torn
½ cup dry white wine
½ medium onion, thinly sliced, lengthwise
1 pint cherry or grape tomatoes, halved lengthwise
1 can artichoke hearts, drained, rinsed, and quartered lengthwise
2 tablespoons olive oil
2 garlic cloves, thinly sliced crosswise
12 ounces whole-wheat spaghetti

In a large pot of boiling salted water, cook the pasta until al dente according to package directions. Drain, reserving 1 cup of pasta water. Return the pasta to pot.

In a large skillet, heat 1 tablespoon of oil over medium-high. Add the onion and garlic, season with salt and pepper, cook, stirring occasionally until browned, 3 to 4 minutes. Add the wine and cook until evaporated, about 2 minutes.

Stir in artichokes and cook until starting to brown for 2 to 3 minutes. Add the olives and half of the tomatoes; cook until tomatoes start to break down, 1 to 2 minutes. Add the pasta to skillet. Stir in remaining tomatoes, oil, cheese, and basil. Thin with reserved pasta water if necessary to coat the spaghetti. Serve with additional cheese.

Mediterranean Pasta

Ingredients
Salt to taste
1 (8 ounce) package linguine pasta
1 pound boneless chicken breast half, cooked and diced
3 slices bacon
1 pound boneless chicken breast half, cooked and diced
1 (14.5 ounce) can peeled and diced tomatoes with juice
1/4 teaspoon dried rosemary
1/3 cup crumbled feta cheese
2/3 cup pitted black olives
1 (6 ounce) can artichoke hearts, drained

Bring a large pot of lightly salted water to a boil. Add the linguine and cook for 8 to 10 minutes or until al dente; drain.

Place the bacon in a large, deep skillet. Cook over medium-high heat until evenly brown. Drain, crumble and set aside.

Season the chicken with salt. Stir chicken with bacon in a large skillet or saucepan. Add tomatoes and rosemary, and simmer for 20 minutes. Stir in feta cheese, olives and artichoke hearts and cook until heated through. Toss with fresh cooked pasta and serve warm. Garnished with extra feta if desired.

Italian Mussels & Pasta

Ingredients
Big pinch of saffron threads (see Note), soaked in 2 tablespoons water or white wine
Freshly ground pepper to taste
Big pinch of crushed red pepper
1/4 cup extra-virgin olive oil
1/4 teaspoon salt
1/4 cup chopped fresh parsley
1 tablespoon finely grated lemon zest (see Tips)
1 15-ounce can crushed tomatoes with basil
¾ cup dry white wine
2 large cloves garlic, chopped
2 pounds mussels, cleaned (see Tips)
8 ounces whole-wheat linguine or spaghetti
3/4 cup dry white wine

Bring a large pot of water to a boil. Cook the pasta according to the package directions. Drain and transfer to a large serving bowl. Cover to keep warm.

Heat oil in a large saucepan over medium heat. Add the garlic and cook, stirring, until it just begins to color for 2 to 3 minutes. Carefully add crushed tomatoes and saffron with soaking liquid (the mixture may splatter) and bring to a simmer. Cook, frequently stirring, until thickened slightly for about 5 minutes.

Bring the mussels and wine to a boil in a Dutch oven (or other large pot) over high heat. Cover, reduce heat to medium and cook until the mussels open for 4 to 6 minutes. Transfer the mussels with a slotted spoon to a large bowl. (Discard any unopened mussels.)

Strain the mussel broth through a fine-mesh sieve into the tomato sauce. Stir in crushed red pepper and simmer over medium heat for 1 minute. Season with salt and pepper. Ladle about half the sauce over the pasta and toss to coat. Divide the pasta among 4 pasta bowls, top with mussels and spoon the remaining sauce over the mussels. Serve topped with parsley and lemon zest.

Mediterranean Baked Penne

Ingredients
1/4 cup dry white wine
1/2 cup fine dry breadcrumbs
1 clove garlic, minced
1 medium eggplant, (about 1 pound), chopped
1 pound dried penne rigate, or rigatoni
1 medium onion, chopped
1 tablespoon extra-virgin olive oil
1 green or red bell pepper, seeded and chopped
1 stalk celery, sliced
1 28-ounce can plum tomatoes, drained and coarsely chopped, juice reserved
1 ½ cups coarsely grated part-skim mozzarella cheese
2 small zucchini, chopped
Salt & freshly ground pepper, to taste
2 large eggs, lightly beaten
2 tablespoons freshly grated Parmesan cheese

Preheat oven to 375°F. Coat a 3-quart baking dish with nonstick spray. Coat the dish with ¼ cup breadcrumbs, tapping out the excess. Put a pot of water on to boil for cooking pasta.

Heat oil in a large nonstick skillet over medium-high heat. Add zucchini, eggplant, bell pepper, onion and celery; cook, stirring occasionally, until tender, about 10 minutes. Add garlic and cook, stirring, for 1 minute more. Add wine and stir until almost evaporated for about 2 minutes.

Add the tomatoes and juice. Bring to a simmer and cook until thickened for 10 to 15 minutes. Season with salt and pepper. Transfer to a large bowl and let cool to room temperature.

Cook penne (or rigatoni) in boiling salted water until al dente for 8 to 10 minutes. Drain and rinse well. Toss the pasta with the vegetable mixture and stir in mozzarella.

Spoon the pasta mixture into prepared baking dish and drizzle eggs evenly over the top. In a small bowl, combine remaining ¼ cup breadcrumbs and Parmesan. Sprinkle evenly over the top.

Bake the pasta until golden, 40-50 minutes. Let stand for 10 minutes.

Bucatini alla Puttanesca

Ingredients
1/8 teaspoon salt plus 1 tablespoon, divided
1 teaspoon finely chopped garlic
1 tablespoon capers, rinsed
1 teaspoon coarsely chopped fresh oregano
2 cups coarsely chopped canned no-salt-added whole peeled tomatoes, with their juice
3 tablespoons extra-virgin olive oil, divided
4 anchovy fillets, chopped
8 black olives, Kalamata or Greek, unpitted
12 ounces bucatini pasta or spaghetti

Combine the anchovies and 2 tablespoons oil in a large saucepan over medium heat. When the anchovies begin to dissolve, add garlic and stir for about 15 seconds. Add the tomatoes and season with 1/8 teaspoon salt; cook until the tomatoes are no longer watery and have separated from the oil for 15 to 20 minutes. Remove from heat.

When the sauce is about halfway done, bring 2 quarts of water to a boil in a large pot. Add the remaining 1 tablespoon salt, then stir in pasta until all the strands are submerged. Cook according to package instructions until just tender.

Cut olives into slivers by slicing the flesh away from the pit. When the pasta is halfway done, return the sauce to medium heat and stir in the olives, capers and oregano.

When the pasta is done, drain well and toss with the sauce, adding the remaining 1 tablespoon oil. Serve at once.

Gnocchi with Zucchini Ribbons & Parsley Brown Butter

Ingredients
Freshly ground pepper, to taste
1/4 teaspoon grated nutmeg
1/2 teaspoon salt
1/2 cup grated Parmesan cheese
1/2 cup chopped fresh parsley
1 pound zucchini, (about 3 small), very thinly sliced lengthwise
1 pint cherry tomatoes, halved
1 pound fresh or frozen gnocchi
2 tablespoons butter
2 medium shallots, chopped
Freshly ground pepper, to taste

Bring a large saucepan of water to a boil. Cook gnocchi until they float for 3 to 5 minutes or according to package directions. Drain.

Melt butter in a large skillet over medium-high heat. Cook until the butter is beginning to brown for about 2 minutes. Add the shallots and zucchini and cook, stirring often, until softened for 2 to 3 minutes.

Add the tomatoes, salt, nutmeg and pepper and continue cooking, stirring often, until the tomatoes are just starting to break down for 1 to 2 minutes. Stir in Parmesan and parsley. Add the gnocchi and toss to coat.

Gnocchi with Tomatoes, Pancetta & Wilted Watercress

Ingredients
1/3 cup freshly grated Parmesan cheese
1/4 teaspoon crushed red pepper
1/4 teaspoon salt
1/2 teaspoon sugar
1 pound gnocchi, (see Shopping Tip)
2 ounces pancetta, chopped
2 large tomatoes, chopped
2 teaspoons red-wine vinegar
3 cloves garlic, minced
4 ounces watercress, tough stems removed, coarsely chopped (6 cups packed)

Put a large pan of water on to boil. Cook the pancetta in a large nonstick skillet over medium heat, stirring occasionally until it begins to brown for 4 to 5 minutes. Add the garlic and cook, stirring for 30 seconds. Add the tomatoes, sugar and crushed red pepper and cook, stirring, until the tomatoes are almost completely broken down, about 5 minutes. Stir in vinegar and salt. Remove from the heat.

Cook the gnocchi in the boiling water until they float for 3 to 5 minutes or according to package directions. Place the watercress in a colander and drain the gnocchi over the watercress, wilting it slightly. Add the gnocchi and watercress to the sauce in the pan; toss to combine. Serve immediately, with Parmesan.

Shrimp & Pesto Pasta

Ingredients
1 pound asparagus, trimmed and cut into 1-inch pieces (about 4 cups)
1/2 cup sliced jarred roasted red peppers
1/4 cup prepared pesto
2 teaspoons extra-virgin olive oil
1 pound raw shrimp, (21-25 per pound), peeled and deveined
1 cup dry white wine
8 ounces whole-wheat fettuccine
Freshly ground pepper, to taste

Bring a large pot of water to a boil. Add fettuccine and cook for 3 minutes less than the package directions specify. Add asparagus and continue cooking until the pasta and asparagus are just tender, about 3 minutes more. Reserving ¼ cup of the cooking water, drain the fettuccine and asparagus and return to the pot. Stir in peppers and pesto. Cover to keep warm.

Heat oil in a large skillet over medium heat. Add shrimp and cook, stirring occasionally, until pink, about 3 minutes. Add wine, increase heat to high and continue cooking until the shrimp are curled and the wine is reduced, about 3 minutes. Add the shrimp and the reserved cooking water to the pasta; toss to coat. Season with pepper and serve immediately.

Mediterranean Baked Penne

Ingredients
1/2 cup fine dry breadcrumbs
1 tablespoon extra-virgin olive oil
1 medium eggplant, (about 1 pound), chopped
1 green or red bell pepper, seeded and chopped
1 medium onion, chopped
1 stalk celery, sliced
1 clove garlic, minced
1/4 cup dry white wine
1 28-ounce can plum tomatoes, drained and coarsely chopped, juice reserved
1 pound dried penne rigate, or rigatoni
1 1/2 cups coarsely grated part-skim mozzarella cheese
2 large eggs, lightly beaten
2 small zucchini, chopped
2 tablespoons freshly grated Parmesan cheese
Salt & freshly ground pepper, to taste

Preheat oven to 375°F. Coat a 3-quart baking dish with nonstick spray. Coat the dish with 1/4 cup breadcrumbs, tapping out the excess. Put a pot of water on to boil for cooking pasta.

Heat oil in a large nonstick skillet over medium-high heat. Add zucchini, eggplant, bell pepper, onion and celery; cook, stirring occasionally, until tender for about 10 minutes. Add garlic and cook, stirring, for 1 minute more. Add the wine and stir until almost evaporated, about 2 minutes. Add tomatoes and juice. Bring to a simmer and cook until thickened for 10 to 15 minutes. Season with salt and pepper. Transfer to a large bowl and let cool to room temperature.

Cook the penne (or rigatoni) in boiling salted water until al dente for 8 to 10 minutes. Drain and rinse well. Toss pasta with the vegetable mixture and stir in mozzarella.

Spoon the pasta mixture into prepared baking dish and drizzle eggs evenly over the top. In a small bowl, combine remaining 1/4 cup breadcrumbs and Parmesan. Sprinkle evenly over the top.

Bake pasta until golden and bubbly for 40 to 50 minutes. Let stand for 10 minutes before serving.

Florentine Ravioli

Ingredients
1 16-ounce bag frozen chopped or whole-leaf spinach
1/8-1/4 teaspoon crushed red pepper
1/4 teaspoon salt
1/2 cup water
1/4 cup freshly grated Parmesan cheese
1 20-ounce package frozen cheese ravioli, or tortellini (4 cups)
4 cloves garlic, minced
6 teaspoons extra-virgin olive oil, divided
1 16-ounce bag frozen chopped or whole-leaf spinach

Bring a large pot of water to a boil; cook ravioli (or tortellini) according to package directions. Heat 2 teaspoons of oil in a large nonstick skillet over medium heat. Add the garlic and cook, stirring, until fragrant for about 30 seconds.

Add salt, crushed red pepper to taste, spinach and water. Cook, stirring frequently, until the spinach has thawed, wilted and heated through for 5 to 7 minutes. Divide among 4 bowls, top with the pasta and drizzle 1 teaspoon of the remaining oil over each portion. Serve immediately with a sprinkle of Parmesan.

Eggplant & Chickpea Baked Pasta

Ingredients
1/2 cup chopped fresh mint or basil, divided
1/2 cup coarse dry whole-wheat breadcrumbs
1 tablespoon extra-virgin olive oil
1 cup crumbled feta cheese
1/2 cup chopped fresh mint or basil, divided
2 tablespoons lemon juice
3 cups Eggplant & Chickpea Stew
8 ounces whole-wheat fusilli

Preheat oven to 350°F. Coat an 8-inch-square (or similar 2-quart) baking dish with cooking spray. Bring a large pot of water to a boil. Cook the pasta according to package directions. Drain and rinse.

Combine breadcrumbs and oil in a small bowl. Toss the pasta with stew, feta, 1/4 cup mint (or basil) and lemon juice in a large bowl. Spread the mixture in the prepared baking dish. Top with the breadcrumb mixture.

Bake until the topping is golden and crispy, about 30 minutes. Sprinkle with the remaining 1/4 cup mint (or basil).

Pasta alle Erbe

Ingredients
1/2 teaspoon crushed red pepper, or to taste
1 pound dry whole-wheat fettuccine
1 cup freshly grated Grana Padano or Parmigiano-Reggiano cheese, plus more for serving
1 cup hot water
1 1/2 pounds quick-cooking leafy greens (about 2 bunches), such as chard, spinach or beet greens
1 1/2 teaspoons kosher salt
2 tablespoons tomato paste
4 plump cloves garlic, peeled and thinly sliced
6 tablespoons extra-virgin olive oil, divided

Put a large pot of water on to boil. Wash the greens, then pat dry. Remove tough stems and coarsely chop the leaves into strips. You should have 10 to 15 cups of chopped greens, depending on the type.

Heat 4 tablespoons of oil in a large skillet over medium-high heat. Add the garlic and cook until starting to color for 30 seconds to 2 minutes. Add the greens a few handfuls at a time, stirring to wilt and fit into the pan. Season with salt and crushed red pepper and stir to coat with oil. Cook, stirring once or twice, until all the greens are wilted, 1 to 3 minutes (or longer, depending on the type of greens you're using).

Whisk water and tomato paste in a bowl. Pour into the skillet and bring to a boil. Cover and adjust the heat to maintain a steady simmer. Cook until the greens are tender and the sauce is reduced slightly, 10 to 15 minutes.

Add the pasta to the boiling water, stirring and separating the strands. Return the water to a boil over high heat and cook the pasta until barely tender for 6 to 8 minutes.

Reserve about 1 cup of the cooking water; drain the pasta. Add the pasta to the greens and toss together for a minute or two until the pasta is coated and fully cooked. If the pasta is too dry, thin the sauce with as much as 1 cup of the reserved pasta water; if too soupy, increase the heat and cook until the sauce thickens.

Remove from the heat. Sprinkle cheese over the pasta; toss well. Drizzle with the remaining 2 tablespoons oil and toss again. Serve immediately, with more cheese, if desired.

Lemon-Garlic Sardine Fettuccine

Ingredients
1/4 cup lemon juice
1/4 cup finely shredded Parmesan cheese
1/2 cup chopped fresh parsley
1/2 teaspoon salt
1 cup fresh breadcrumbs, preferably whole-wheat
1/4 cup lemon juice
1 teaspoon freshly ground pepper
2 3- to 4-ounce cans boneless, skinless sardines, preferably in tomato sauce, flaked
4 tablespoons extra-virgin olive oil, divided
4 cloves garlic, minced
8 ounces whole-wheat fettuccine

Bring a large pot of water to a boil. Cook the pasta until just tender for 8 to 10 minutes or according to package directions. Drain.

Heat 2 tablespoons of oil in a small nonstick skillet over medium heat. Add the garlic and cook, stirring, until fragrant and sizzling but not brown about 20 seconds. Transfer the garlic and oil to a large bowl.

Heat the remaining 2 tablespoons oil in the pan over medium heat. Add breadcrumbs and cook, stirring, until crispy and golden brown, 5 to 6 minutes. Transfer to a plate.

Whisk lemon juice, pepper and salt into the garlic oil. Add the pasta to the bowl along with sardines, parsley and Parmesan. Gently stir to combine. Serve sprinkled with the breadcrumbs.

Inside-Out Lasagna

Ingredients
1/4 teaspoon freshly ground pepper
1/2 teaspoon crushed red pepper (optional)
1/2 teaspoon salt
3/4 cup part-skim ricotta cheese
1 tablespoon extra-virgin olive oil
1 onion, chopped
3 cloves garlic, sliced
8 ounces sliced white mushrooms (about 3 1/2 cups)
8 cups baby spinach
8 ounces whole-wheat rotini or fusilli

Bring a large pot of water to a boil. Add pasta; cook until just tender, 8 to 10 minutes or according to package directions. Drain and transfer to a large bowl.

Heat oil in a large nonstick skillet over medium heat. Add the onion and garlic and cook, stirring, until soft and beginning to brown, about 3 minutes. Add mushrooms, salt and pepper and cook, stirring, until the mushrooms release their liquid, 4 to 6 minutes.

Add tomatoes, spinach and crushed red pepper (if using). Increase heat to medium-high; cook, stirring once halfway through, until the spinach is wilted, about 4 minutes.

Toss the sauce with the pasta and divide among 4 bowls. Dollop each serving with 3 tablespoons of ricotta.

Creamy Garlic Pasta with Shrimp & Vegetables

Ingredients
1/4 cup toasted pine nuts (optional)
1/4 cup chopped flat-leaf parsley
1/2 teaspoon freshly ground pepper
1 1/4 teaspoons kosher salt
1 1/2 cups nonfat or low-fat plain yogurt
1 tablespoon extra-virgin olive oil
1 bunch asparagus, trimmed and thinly sliced
1 large red bell pepper, thinly sliced
1 cup fresh or frozen peas
3 tablespoons lemon juice
3 cloves garlic, chopped
6 ounces whole-wheat spaghetti
12 ounces peeled and deveined raw shrimp, cut into 1-inch pieces

Bring a large pot of water to a boil. Add spaghetti and cook 2 minutes less than package directions. Add shrimp, asparagus, bell pepper and peas and cook until the pasta is tender and the shrimp are cooked, 2 to 4 minutes more. Drain well.

Mash garlic and salt in a large bowl until a paste forms. Whisk in yogurt, parsley, lemon juice, oil and pepper. Add the pasta mixture and toss to coat. Serve sprinkled with pine nuts (if using).

Fusilli with Italian Sausage & Arugula

Ingredients
1/8 teaspoon salt
1/4 cup finely shredded Pecorino Romano, or Parmesan cheese
1/2 cup halved cherry tomatoes
1 teaspoon freshly ground pepper
2 cloves garlic, chopped
2 teaspoons extra-virgin olive oil
4 ounces whole-wheat pasta, such as shells or fusilli
4 ounces hot Italian turkey sausage, removed from casing
4 cups arugula, or baby spinach

Bring a large pot of water to a boil. Cook pasta for 8 to 10 minutes or according to package directions. Cook sausage in a large nonstick skillet over medium-high heat, breaking it into small pieces with a wooden spoon, until cooked through, 2 to 4 minutes.

Stir in garlic, arugula (or spinach) and tomatoes. Cook, stirring often, until the greens wilt and the tomatoes begin to break down, 1 to 2 minutes. Remove from the heat; cover and keep warm.

Combine the cheese, pepper and salt in a large bowl. Measure out 2 tablespoons of the cooking liquid; drain the pasta. Whisk the cooking liquid and oil into the cheese mixture; add the pasta and toss to combine. Serve the pasta topped with the sausage-arugula mixture.

Zucchini, Fennel & White Bean Pasta

Ingredients
1/4 teaspoon salt
1/4 cup fresh mint leaves
3/4 cup crumbled hard, aged goat cheese, or fresh goat cheese
1 cup cooked cannellini beans, plus 1/2 cup bean-cooking liquid, pasta-cooking liquid or water
1 large fennel bulb, trimmed
2 cloves garlic, finely chopped
2 medium zucchini
2 plum tomatoes, diced
3 tablespoons extra-virgin olive oil, divided
8 ounces (2 cups) whole-wheat penne or similar short pasta
2 cloves garlic, finely chopped
Freshly ground pepper to taste

Preheat oven to 400°F. Cut the fennel bulb in half lengthwise and then slice lengthwise into 1/2-inch-thick wedges. Quarter zucchini lengthwise. Toss the fennel and zucchini with 1 tablespoon of oil and salt. Arrange in a single layer on a large baking sheet. Roast, turning once, until soft and beginning to brown for about 20 minutes.

Bring a large pot of water to a boil. Add pasta; cook until just tender, 8 to 10 minutes or according to package directions. Heat the remaining 2 tablespoons of oil in a large skillet over medium heat. Add the garlic and cook, stirring, for 30 seconds. Remove from the heat.

When the vegetables are cool enough to handle, coarsely chop. Add the vegetables, beans and bean-cooking liquid (or other liquid) to the pan with the garlic and place over medium-low heat. Drain the pasta and immediately add it to the pan. Toss thoroughly and add tomatoes; toss until just warm. Remove from the heat and stir in cheese and mint. Season with pepper.

Mediterranean Summer Pasta with Salsa Cruda

Ingredients
1/3 cup olive oil
1/2 cup flavorful pitted olives, lightly chopped
1 teaspoon red pepper flakes
1 clove garlic, smashed
1 teaspoon orange zest
2 tablespoons capers
2 ripe tomatoes, seeded and chopped
2 to 3 tablespoons chopped fresh mint
12 ounces angel hair pasta
Kosher salt and freshly cracked pepper
Parmesan, for grating

In a large pasta serving bowl, mix together the olives, tomatoes, mint, capers, garlic, red pepper flakes, orange zest and olive oil. Season with salt and freshly cracked pepper. Stir and lightly press the ingredients with the back of the spoon to incorporate flavors. Let it sit for at least 30 minutes or for a day.

Just before serving, cook the angel hair pasta in salted boiling water according to package instructions. Remove the garlic clove from the pasta sauce. Drain the pasta and while still steaming hot, place the pasta on top of the cold sauce. Let it sit for a minute before tossing the pasta. Top with grated Parmesan and serve.

Bean Bolognese

Ingredients
1 14-ounce can salad beans, (see Shopping Tip) or other beans, rinsed, divided
1 bay leaf
1 small onion, chopped
1/2 cup chopped carrot
1/2 teaspoon salt
1/4 cup chopped celery
2 tablespoons extra-virgin olive oil
4 cloves garlic, chopped
1/2 cup white wine
1 14-ounce can diced tomatoes
1/4 cup chopped fresh parsley, divided
8 ounces whole-wheat fettuccine
1/2 cup freshly grated Parmesan cheese
8 ounces whole-wheat fettuccine

Put a large pot of water on to boil. Mash 1/2 cup beans in a small bowl with a fork. Heat the oil in a medium saucepan over medium heat. Add the onion, carrot, celery and salt; cover and cook, stirring occasionally, until softened for about 10 minutes. Add the garlic and bay leaf; cook, stirring, until fragrant for about 15 seconds. Add the wine; increase heat to high and boil until most of the liquid evaporates, 3 to 4 minutes.

Add the tomatoes and their juices, 2 tablespoons parsley and the mashed beans. Bring to a lively simmer and cook, stirring occasionally, until thickened, about 6 minutes. Add the remaining whole beans; cook, stirring occasionally, until heated through, 1 to 2 minutes more.

Meanwhile, cook the pasta in the boiling water until just tender for about 9 minutes or according to package directions. Drain. Divide the pasta among 4 bowls. Discard the bay leaf and top the pasta with the sauce; sprinkle with Parmesan and the remaining parsley.

Mediterranean Pasta with Lamb Meatballs

Ingredients
Spice mix, divided, recipe follows
3/4 cup fat free, low-sodium chicken stock
1 1/2 pounds ground lamb
1 teaspoon ground cinnamon
1 teaspoon freshly ground black pepper
1 teaspoon kosher salt, divided
1 cup feta cheese, divided
2 tablespoons olive oil
2 green onions, finely sliced
2 shallots, minced
2 (28-ounce) cans diced tomatoes
2 tablespoons chopped fresh parsley leaves
5 cloves garlic, minced, divided
12 ounces spaghetti
15 mini unsalted matzoh crackers, ground into crumbs

Spice mix:
1/2 teaspoon dried thyme
1/2 teaspoon dried marjoram
1 teaspoon dried rosemary
1 teaspoon cumin seeds
1 1/2 teaspoons coriander seeds
1 1/2 teaspoons granulated onion
1 1/2 teaspoons dried oregano

Preheat oven to 350 degrees F. For meatballs: combine lamb, 2 teaspoons of the spice mix, the ground matzoh crackers, 2 cloves garlic, 1/2 teaspoon salt and 3/4 cup feta cheese. Mix until combined but do not over mix.

Divide into 16 equal portions; shape into meatballs. Place meatballs on rack over cookie sheet so grease will drain from meatballs while cooking; bake 20 minutes.

For sauce: heat olive oil in saucepan over medium heat and add shallots and remaining garlic. Cook until limp and translucent for 2 to 3 minutes. Add the tomatoes, remainder of spice mix, cinnamon, pepper, remainder of the salt, chicken stock, and parsley. Bring to boil; reduce to a simmer and cook until thick, about 15 minutes, stirring occasionally.

Cook pasta according to package directions and drain.

To cooked sauce, add sliced green onion and meatballs stirring gently to coat. Serve meatballs with sauce over pasta and garnish with remaining feta cheese.

Spice mix: In a blender or coffee grinder pulse coriander, rosemary, thyme, cumin, marjoram, oregano, and onion until a fine consistency.

WRAPS

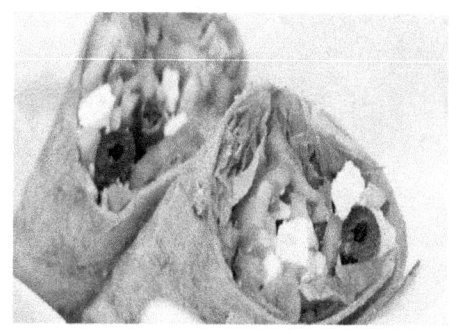

Mediterranean Shrimp Wraps

Ingredients
1 cup baby spinach leaves
4 tablespoons prepared basil pesto
4 flour tortillas, regular or flavored
1 (14-ounce) can artichoke hearts, drained and chopped
1/2 cup diced sun-dried tomatoes
Cooked shrimp, cut into 1/2-inch pieces (about 1 to 1 1/2 cups total)

Spread pesto on 1 side of tortillas. Top with spinach, shrimp, artichoke hearts, and sun-dried tomatoes and roll up.

Mediterranean Wrap

Ingredients
3/4 cup chopped tomato
1 tablespoon diced red onion
1 tablespoon chopped fresh cilantro
1 teaspoon lime juice
1 cup chopped red bell pepper
1/4 cup (1 ounce) crumbled feta cheese
1/8 teaspoon salt
1 garlic clove, minced
1 cup hot cooked jasmine or long-grain rice
2 tablespoons chopped fresh or 2 teaspoons dried basil
3/4 cup chopped tomato
3/4 cup diced zucchini
3/4 cup diced yellow squash
1/4 cup diced red onion
2 tablespoons balsamic vinegar
2 teaspoons olive oil
4 (8-inch) fat-free flour tortillas

Preheat broiler. Combine the first 6 ingredients in a bowl and set aside. Combine rice and basil; set aside.

Arrange bell pepper, zucchini, yellow squash, and 1/4 cup red onion in a single layer on a baking sheet. Broil for 12 minutes or until the vegetables are browned; spoon into a large bowl. Drizzle vinegar and oil over vegetables; toss to coat.

Warm tortillas according to package directions. Spoon 1/4 cup of rice mixture down center of each tortilla. Top each with 1/2 cup roasted vegetables, 2 tablespoons tomato mixture, and 1 tablespoon cheese; roll up.

Mediterranean Spinach Turkey Wrap

Ingredients
1/2 cup Kraft cream cheese with chives and onions
1/2 cup feta cheese, crumbled (the sharper the better)
1/4 black olives
1/4 teaspoon oregano
1 cup loosely packed thoroughly washed spinach leaves
4 ounces smoked turkey, thinly sliced
32 inches flour tortillas (spinach flavored preferably)

Chop up olives. Combine cream cheese, feta cheese, olives and oregano in bowl and mix. Evenly spread the mixture over entire tortilla.

Place the turkey over the cream cheese mixture on half of each tortilla. Place the spinach leaves on top of turkey. To assemble, just start with the side that is topped with the turkey and roll up tightly. Wrap each sandwich with saran wrap. Refrigerate wraps for at least 1 hour.

Before serving, unwrap, and trim of ends of each roll. Cut wraps slightly diagonal into 3 sections.

Mediterranean Veggie Wrap

Ingredients
1/4 cup fresh parsley, chopped
1 soft cracker bread, halved (Lavosh) or 1 large flour tortilla
1 small cucumber, thinly sliced
1 small tomatoes, seeded and chopped
1 ounce feta cheese, crumbled
4 ounces hummus
8 ripe olives, sliced

Spread hummus on the bread to within 1/2 inch of the edge.
Add parsley, cucumber, olives, tomato, and cheese on top of hummus.
Roll up and serve.

Greek Isles Wrap

Ingredients
1/4 cup Mayonnaise
1 cucumber, sliced
1 container (4 oz.) crumbled feta cheese
1 cup pitted Kalamata olives
4 leaves romaine lettuce
4 (8-inch) plain or pesto & garlic flavored tortillas
8 cherry tomatoes, quartered (about 1/2 cup)
Lemon juice or distilled white vinegar
Dried oregano leaves, crushed (optional)

Spread Hellmann's® or Best Foods® Real Mayonnaise generously on tortillas. Layer lettuce, cucumber, cheese, olives and tomatoes down center of each tortilla. Sprinkle with lemon juice and oregano. Roll and fold the filled tortillas.

Tempeh Greek Salad Wraps

Ingredients
1/4 tsp salt
1/4 cup feta cheese crumbles ? Tasty tip
1/4 tsp ground black pepper (freshly)
1/2 tsp paprika
1 garlic cloves (minced)
1 cup water
1 cup romaine lettuce (shredded)
1 tsp grated lemon zest
1 1/2 tsps Italian seasoning (dried, divided)
2 tbsps plain low-fat yogurt
2 tbsps plain low-fat yogurt
2 tbsps olive oil (divided)
2 cups baby spinach (bagged)
3 tbsps lemon juice (divided)
8 ozs tempeh (organic, cut into 24 pieces)
2/3 cup cherry tomatoes (sliced)
2/3 cup english cucumber (sliced)
1/4 cup feta cheese crumbles
1/4 tsp ground black pepper (freshly)
4 whole wheat tortillas

Heat a 10-inch skillet over medium-high heat. Add 1 tablespoon oil; swirl to coat. Add tempeh; sauté 4 minutes or until lightly browned, turning once. Add 1 cup water and 2 tablespoons juice to pan; reduce heat to medium, and simmer 10 minutes, turning once.

Combine 2 tablespoons yogurt, 1/2 teaspoon Italian seasoning, and the next 4 ingredients (through garlic) in a small bowl.

Combine 1 tablespoon olive oil, 1 tablespoon lemon juice, 1 teaspoon Italian seasoning, spinach, and next 5 ingredients in a bowl.

Warm tortillas according to the package directions. Spread 2 teaspoons yogurt mixture over each tortilla. Top each tortilla with 3/4 cup spinach mixture and 6 pieces tempeh; roll up. Cut each rolled tortilla in half crosswise.

Mediterranean Chickpea and Feta Salad Wrap with Creamy Greek Dressing

Ingredients
Pinch of garlic powder
Salt and pepper to taste
a handful of greens
A few thin slices of red onion
1/4 teaspoon oregano
1/4 cup cooked chickpeas, drained and rinsed
1/4 cup chopped cucumber
1/4 cup chopped feta cheese
1/4 cup chopped tomato
1/4 cup chopped pitted olives (optional) 2 tablespoons Greek yogurt
1 teaspoon red wine vinegar
1 tablespoon olive oil
1 whole wheat tortilla wrap
2 tablespoons Greek yogurt

In a medium mixing bowl, whisk together yogurt, vinegar, olive oil, oregano, garlic powder, salt, and pepper. Taste and adjust seasonings if needed.

Add remaining ingredients except tortilla; mix to coat evenly in dressing.

Add mixture to the tortilla, wrap like a burrito.

Quinoa Greek Salad Lettuce Wraps

Ingredients
For the Vinaigrette:
1 ½ tablespoons freshly squeezed lemon juice
1/2 tablespoon red wine vinegar
1/4 teaspoon dried oregano
1 teaspoon minced garlic
2 tablespoons extra virgin olive oil
kosher salt and black pepper, to taste

For the Quinoa:
½ cup quinoa, rinsed and drained
kosher salt and pepper
1 cup grape tomatoes, halved
½ cup pitted kalamata olives, roughly chopped
½ cup red onion, finely chopped
1 cup cucumber, chopped
1 pepperoncini pepper, stem removed and finely chopped (optional)
crumbled feta cheese, for sprinkling on top
romaine lettuce hearts, leaves separated to make long, narrow lettuce cups

In a small bowl, whisk together the lemon juice, vinegar, oregano, garlic, olive oil, and salt and pepper to taste. Cover and refrigerate.

To a small saucepan over medium-high heat, add the rinsed quinoa, 1 cup of water, and salt and pepper. Cover and bring to a boil. Reduce heat to low and simmer the quinoa for 12-15 minutes until quinoa is cooked and water is absorbed. Remove from the heat, remove the lid and fluff quinoa with a fork, allowing the quinoa to cool.

In the meantime, add to a mixing bowl the tomatoes, olives, red onion, cucumber, and pepper (if using). Fold in the cooled quinoa. Drizzle with the prepared vinaigrette and toss to combine. Refrigerate the salad for at least one hour before serving.

To assemble the lettuce wraps: just prior to serving, place the romaine lettuce cups onto a work surface. Using a small spoon, carefully scoop the Greek quinoa salad into the cups. Sprinkle each lettuce wrap with a generous amount of feta cheese. Transfer the lettuce wraps to a serving plate. Serve promptly. Recipe is easily doubled.

Mediterranean Pesto Wrap

Ingredients
1/4 of an avocado, sliced
1 tablespoon roughly chopped cilantro
1 small cucumber, cut into thin spears
1 piece lavash bread (or your favorite wrap or pita)
2-4 tablespoons garlic hummus
2 tablespoons basil pesto
4 falafel (or one of the protein replacements from above!)
5-8 kalamata olives, pitted and sliced
handful of mixed greens
sprinkle of hot sauce (optional, but recommended)

Heat your oven on low to prepare to heat your lavash bread.
Bake/ heat your falafel or prepare your protein of choice. While your protein cooks, cut up your cucumbers, onions, avocado, olives, and cilantro.

Place your lavash bread in the oven for a minute to warm it up. Heat it too long and the wrap will become too hard to fold and wrap easily, so just let it get warm, then pull it. Once you have pulled it, lay it on a work surface, like a large cutting board. Spread hummus evenly around the middle of the lavash.

Top with falafel, then pesto. Arrange cucumber, onion, & avocado around falafel width-wise (like shown below). Sprinkle with sliced olives, chopped cilantro, and hot sauce. Finally, toss on a hearty handful of greens.

Starting at one end of the lavash bread, begin to roll the wrap up away from you, tucking the innards in to the bread under as you roll to form a tight wrap, which help keep your ingredients in.

If you prefer to tuck the ends in around the roll, more 'burrito-style'- go for it. Once it's rolled up tight, use a serrated knife to slice the wrap in half at a slight angle. Serve, enjoy!

Mediterranean Snack Wrap

Ingredients
1 piece whole wheat lavash bread, lightly toasted
1 pinch freshly ground black pepper
1 tablespoon chopped, toasted walnuts
1-2 tablespoons fig butter or preserves
2 ounces French or Greek feta in brine

Toast walnut pieces and set aside to cool. Gently toast whole wheat lavash bread or some other middle eastern flatbread.

Spread fig butter on the warm bread, sprinkle over walnuts and crush in pieces of feta

ADDITIONAL RESOURCES

Please point your web browser to **www.plaid-enterprises.com** for more related resources, my full bibliography and to grab your FREE book!

Grab Your Free 'Drop 10 Pounds in 7 Days' Report at:
http://www.plaid-enterprises.com/mediterranean

www.ingramcontent.com/pod-product-compliance
Lightning Source LLC
Chambersburg PA
CBHW070323290526
45791CB00003B/1239